Author

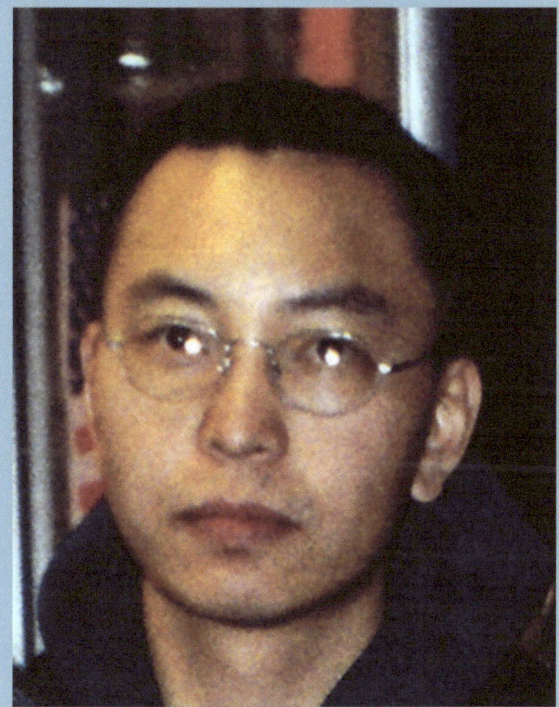

I've been a street body workout pioneer for over 20 years. During that time, I've have conditioned amateur wrestling champions and street athletes which they utilize my methods in their personal and professional life.

Water Kung Fu was developed utilizing my life's experience in body street exercises, US Naval Aircrew training and cross training with various special ops units. All these proven goodies are put together in a healing training regiment.

My goals of this 1st volume are two fold. One, introduce the world to Water Kung Fu. Two, to make available the pool design so any community in the world can build their own Water Kung Fu pool park in the open or indoors.

I'm available on individual and group consultation of no more than 5 at a time. I can be contacted at taisondua@yahoo.com. I recommend a minimum of 2 hours of consultation with me to get the full benefits of Water Kung Fu for technique and safety reasons.

Table of Contents

Author i

Table of Contents ii

Introduction 1, 2

Pool Design 3

PreStretch, PostStretch 4

Phase 1 5

Phase 2 6

Phase 3 7

Make It Rain 8

Chi Kick 9

Chi Sweep Kick 10

Hand Oar 11

Flower 12

Out of Trouble 13

Hand Oar Muay Thai Kick 14

Water for Heaven 15

Hug and Throw 16

Chi Float 17

Chi Sit-up 18

Making a Rainbow 19

Over the Rainbow 20

Riding the Rainbow 21

Chi Engine 22

Water Kung Fu was developed to maximize body and mind performance without damage to the joints.

Water Kung Fu has 15 moves. Each move is done in 7 minute intervals to the best of one's ability with 2 minutes cool down and 1 minute to hydrate. The only exception is the Chi Float at the end of phase 2 and 3 that requires 30 minutes. The Chi Float is exercise, cool down and meditation all in one. All moves that has contact with the pool bottom will be moving forward as you do them. Prestretch and poststretch are your standard swimming stretches with the addition of an ankle extension stretch.

Water Kung Fu is ideally practiced outside in a customized pool with adjustable height platform. The floor of the pool is to be flat and none abrasive. The pool is to be constructed with heavy duty hard wood and stainless steel. The customized pool should be at least 6 feet wide by 30 feet long for each person. The height should be adjustable between 2 to 6 feet deep. (Pool Desigh) The pool should have a solid stainless metal handle bar at one end and an adjustable 2 to 7 feet above water level rotating solid stainless metal bar in the middle. This design will allow for different people to do all the different moves.

If you do not have access to a custom pool near you, you can still finish the 1st 2 phases at your local pool.

There's some basic guidelines you should take to be successful with the program. 1st is a good workout diet. 2nd is 8 hours of sleep. 3rd is a calm and clear mind.

If you are trying to lose weight, then follow this diet...

Workout day, drink 16 ounces of hot green tea and 16 ounces of hot water 1 hour before workout. After the workout, drink 16 ounces of coconut juice with a normal healthy lunch. The rest of the day eat and drink normal healthy food. Make sure you get 8 hours of sleep. Earplugs are great for this. Go to a safety gear shop or get boxes of them online.

None workout day, drink 16 ounces of hot green tea and 16 ounces of hot water and eat a light protein breakfast. For the rest of the day, eat light snacks of fruit, vegitable and nuts and drink a lot of hot water. Make sure you get your 8 hours of sleep. You should get close to your ideal weight in about 3 months just doing the 1st 2 phases and following this diet.

There are 3 phases consisting of different combination of moves. Phase 1 is to build your core to get you to the proper weight with the right diet and sleep which require (3) 1 hour of your time each week. Phase 2 is to build your stamina, athleticism, breathing technique and a meditative mind. This phase require (3) 1.5 hour per week. Phase 3 is combining phase 2 with strength training and should be done with a custom pool. This phase require (3) 2 hours per week. You can do phase 2 then substitute the strength portion with standard weights and body weight exercises, but the reason to do phase 3 in a custom pool is that it's safer, more fun and less impact on your body so you have better results.

It takes about 2 months to progress from 1 phase to the next. Do which ever phase you are comfortable with for your condition. I hope you will continue using Water Kung Fu as one of your life long conditioning tools. Always consult with your physician before you begin a new workout routine.

Pool Design

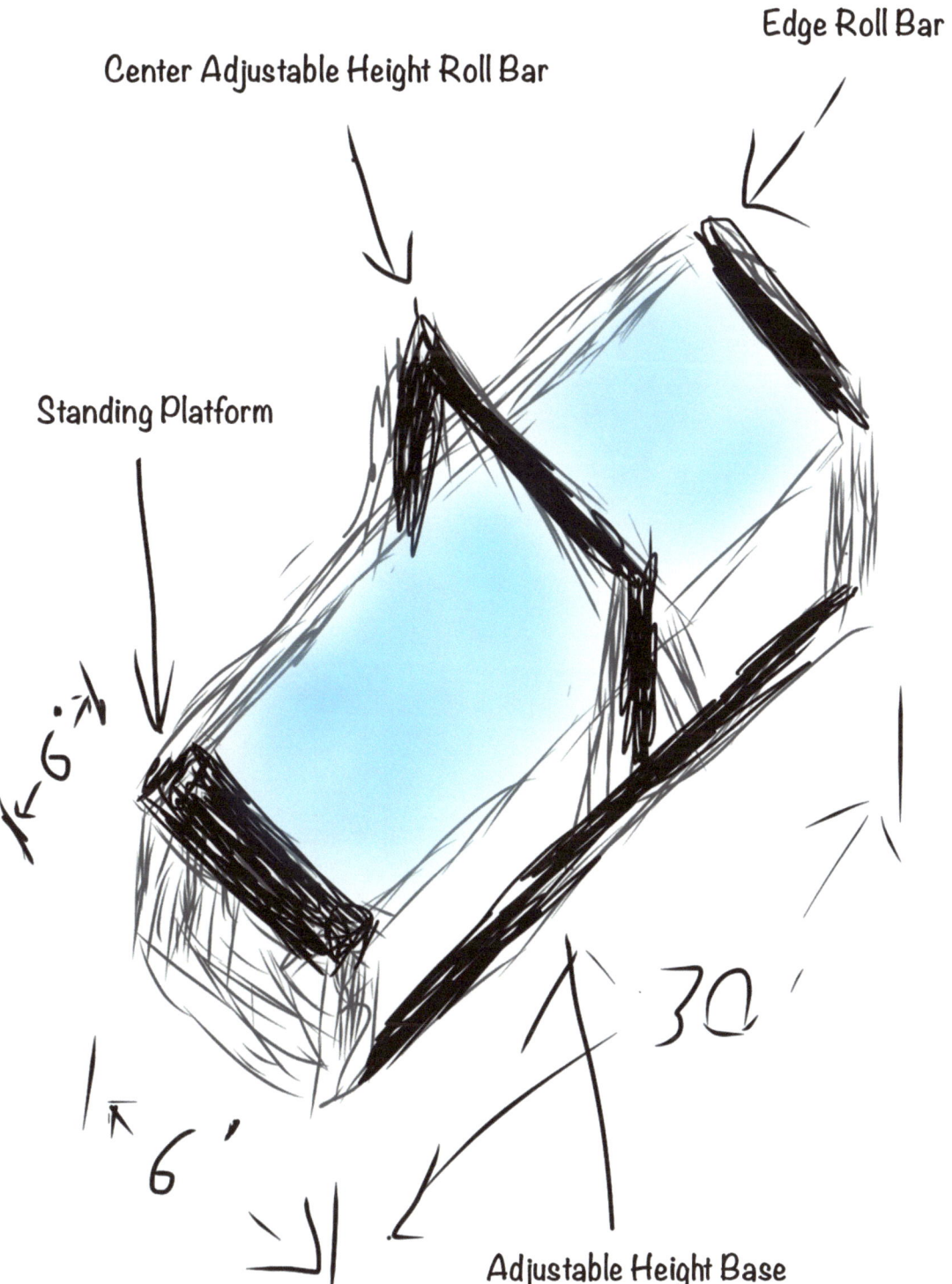

Center Adjustable Height Roll Bar

Edge Roll Bar

Standing Platform

Adjustable Height Base

6'

6'

30'

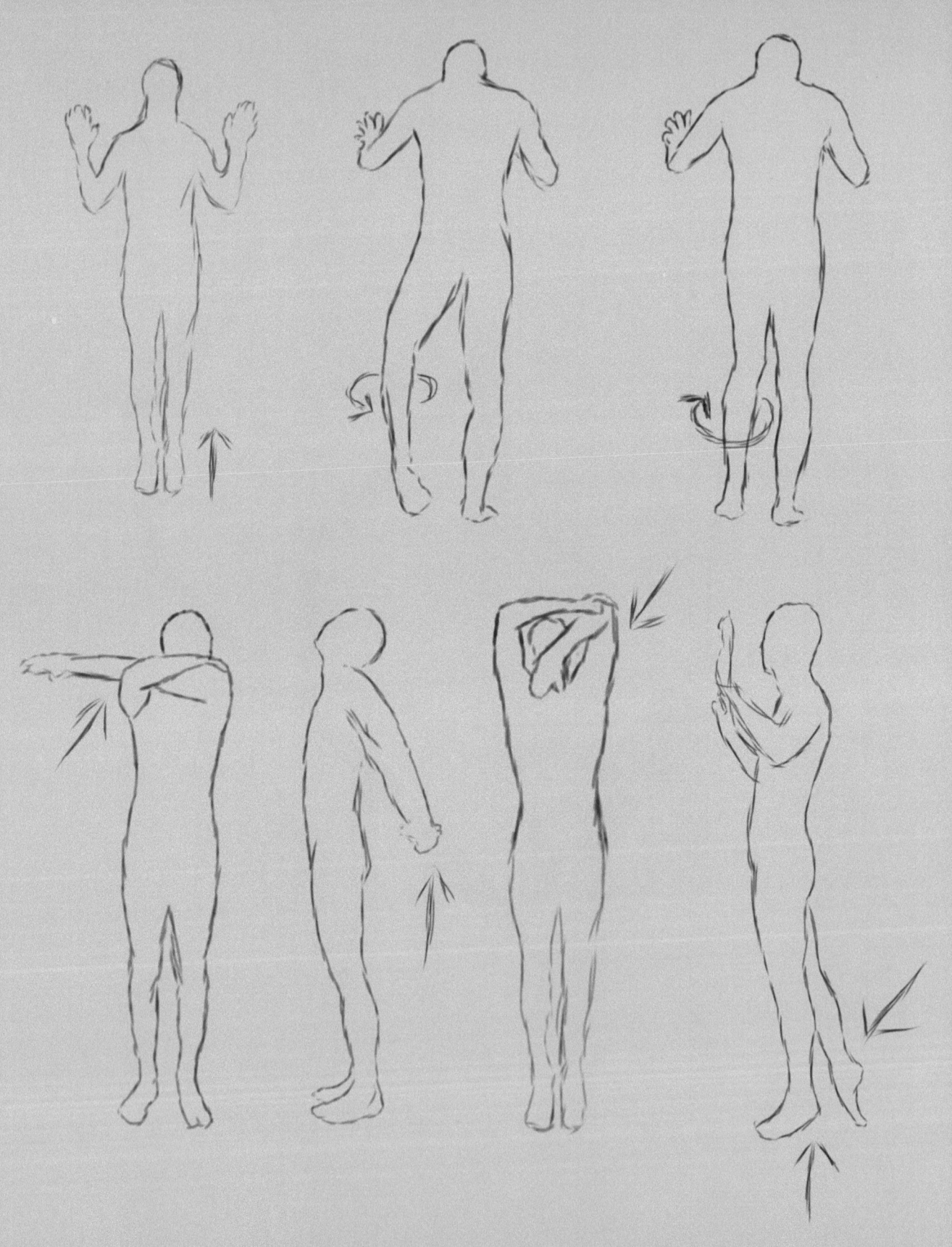

PreStretch

Make It Rain
Chi Kick
Chi Sweep Kick
Hand Oar
Flower

PostStretch

PreStretch

Chi Kick
Chi Sweep Kick
Out of Trouble
Hand Oar Muay Thai Kick
Water for Heaven
Hug and Throw
Chi Float

PostStretch

PreStretch

Chi Kick
Chi Sweep Kick
Out of Trouble
Hand Oar Muay Thai Kick
Chi Sit-up
Making a Rainbow
Over the Rainbow
Riding the Rainbow
Chi Engine
Chi Float

PostStretch

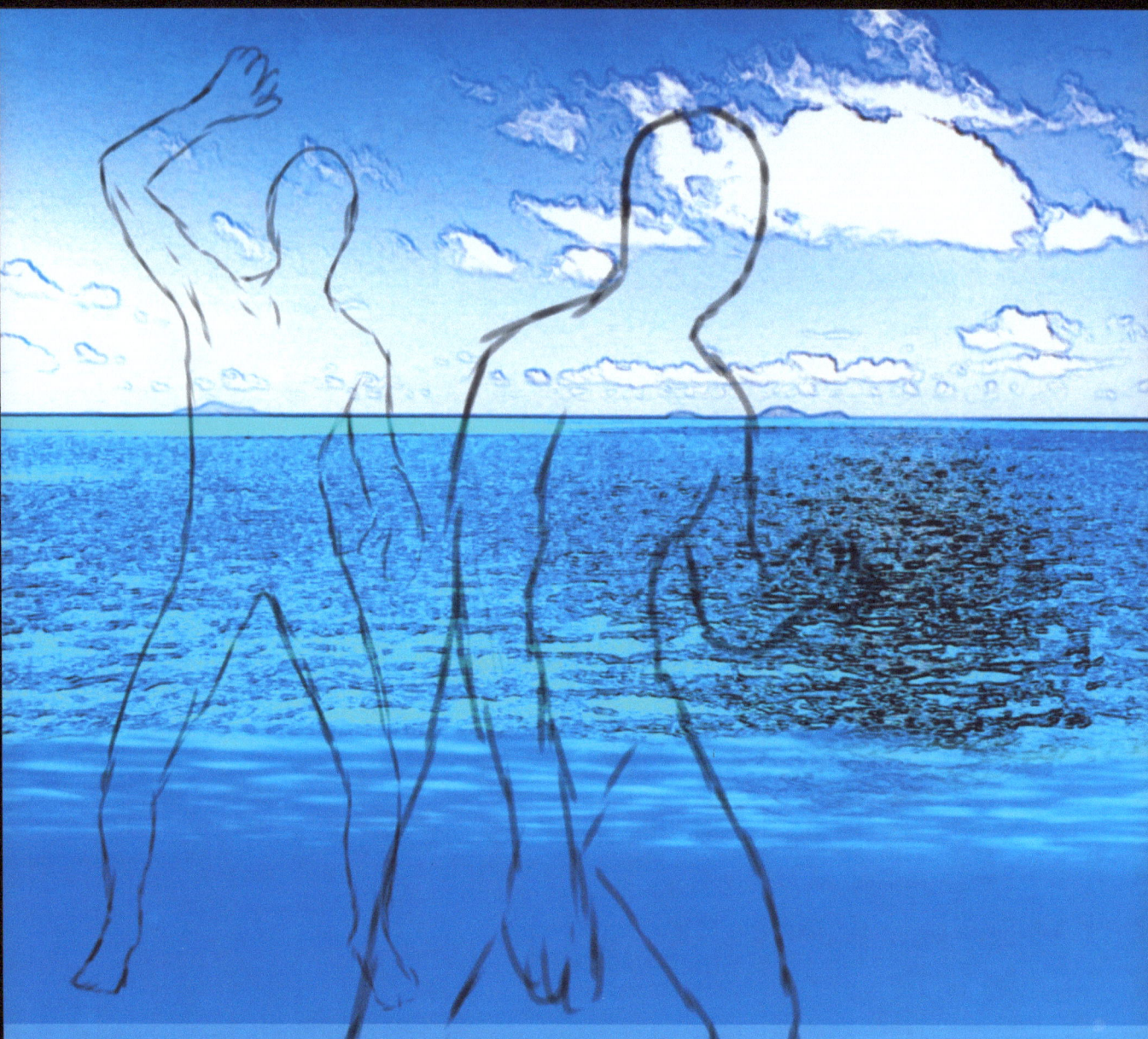

Standing wide in waist deep water,
strike the water with your hands and arms.
Alternate sides as you strike the water.
Do this to release all stress, make it look like rain
and clear your mind to start your phase.

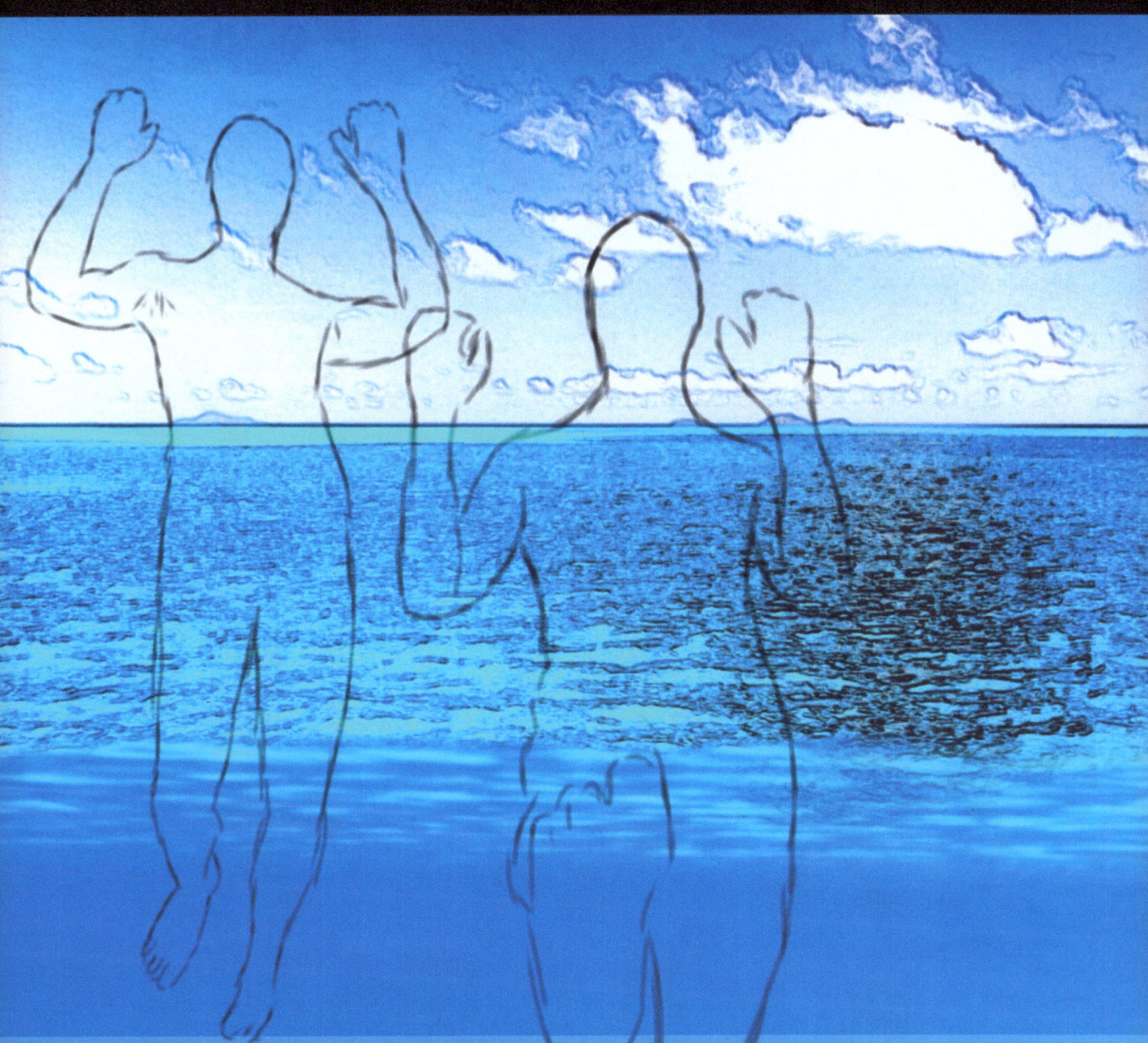

Water at liver level. Arms at shoulder height, do a one legged kick with your stomach muscles and leaning back straight at about 30 degrees. Alternate legs. The purpose of this move is to generate as much wave from your stomach muscles as you can.

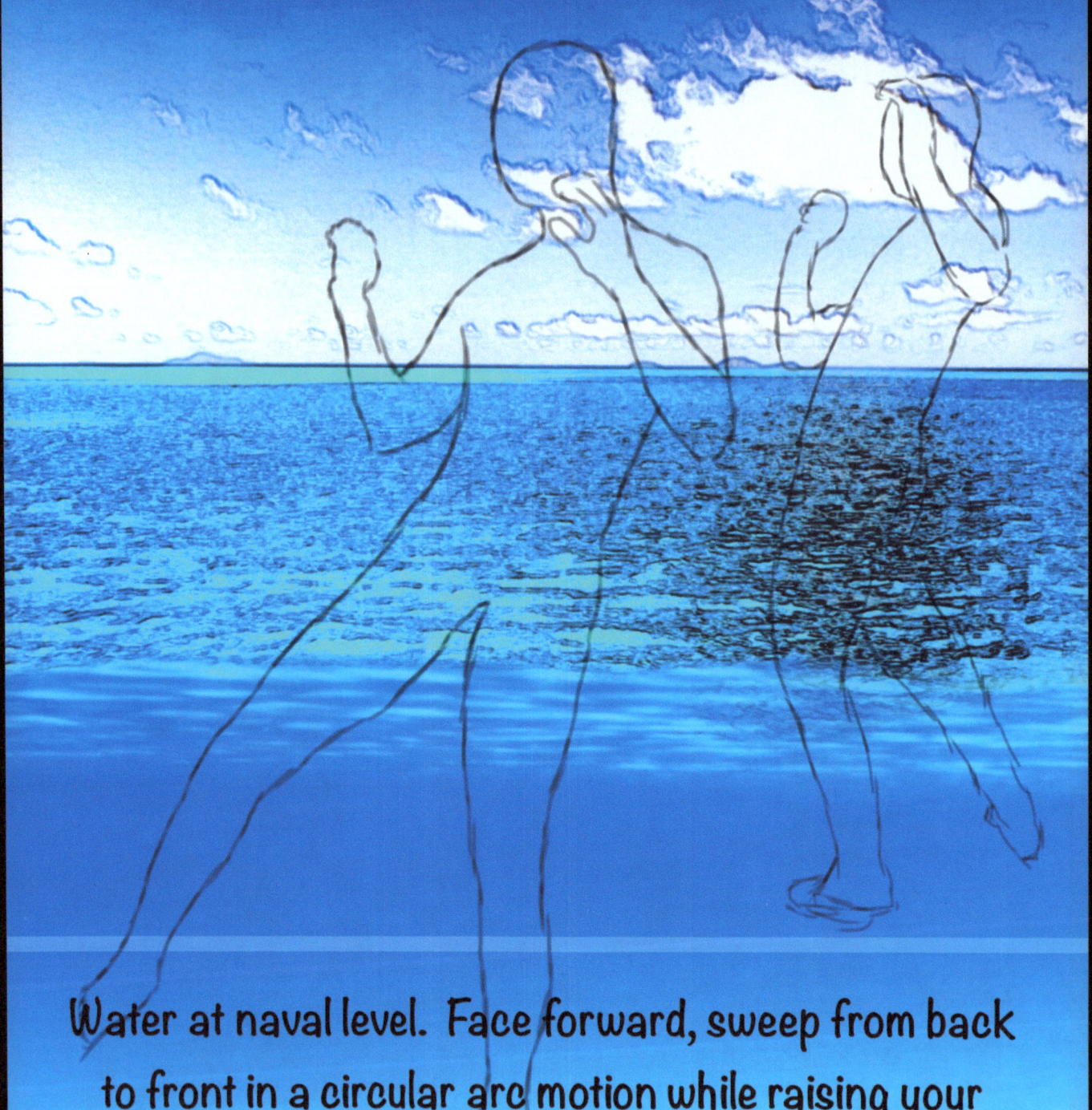

Water at naval level. Face forward, sweep from back to front in a circular arc motion while raising your supporting ankle like a ballet dancer. End each sweep using your side waist muscles. Alternate Legs.

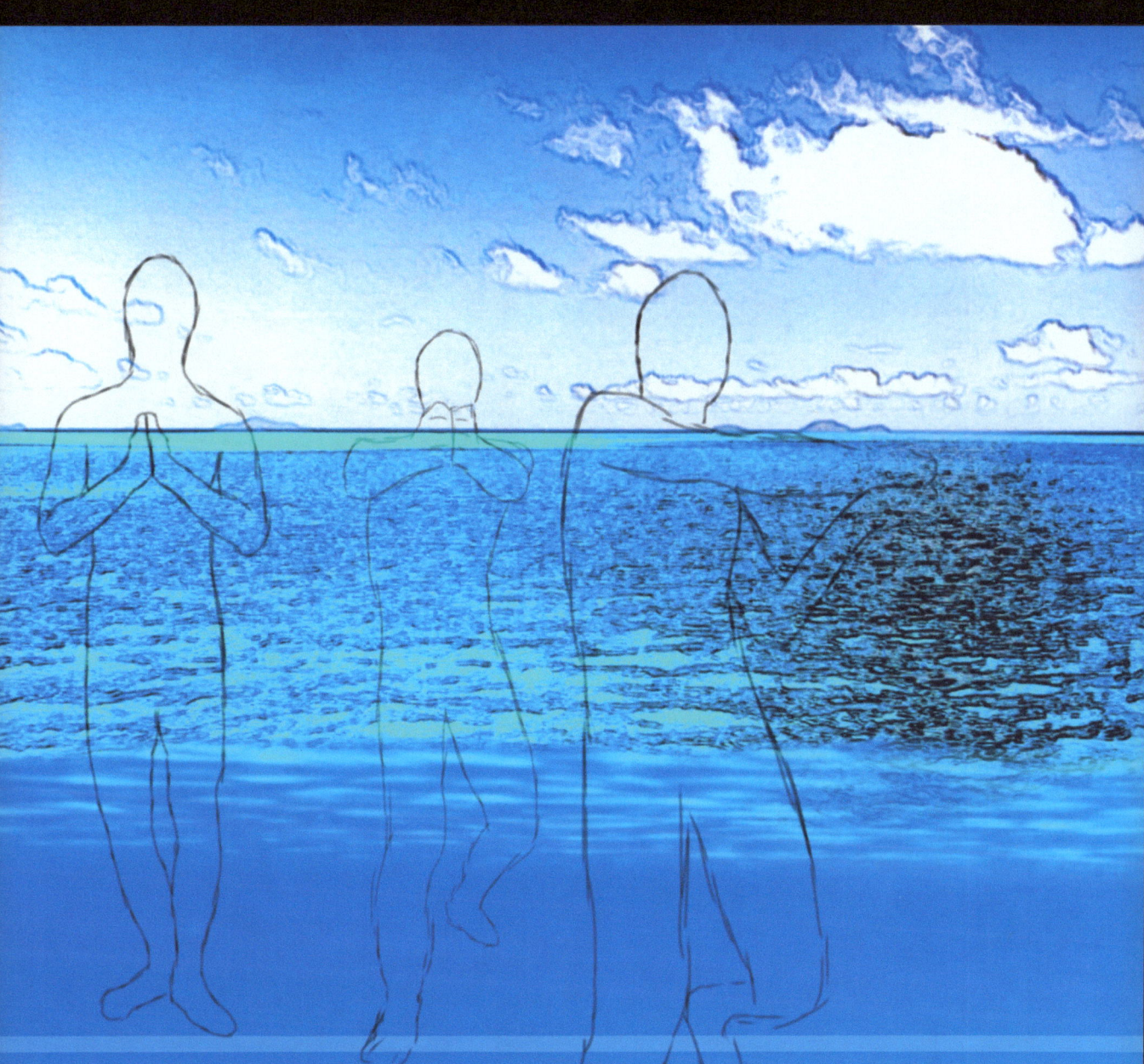

Water at chest level. Holding your hands together at your chest, push straight in front of you, swing to one side to move yourself forward. Repeat on other side.

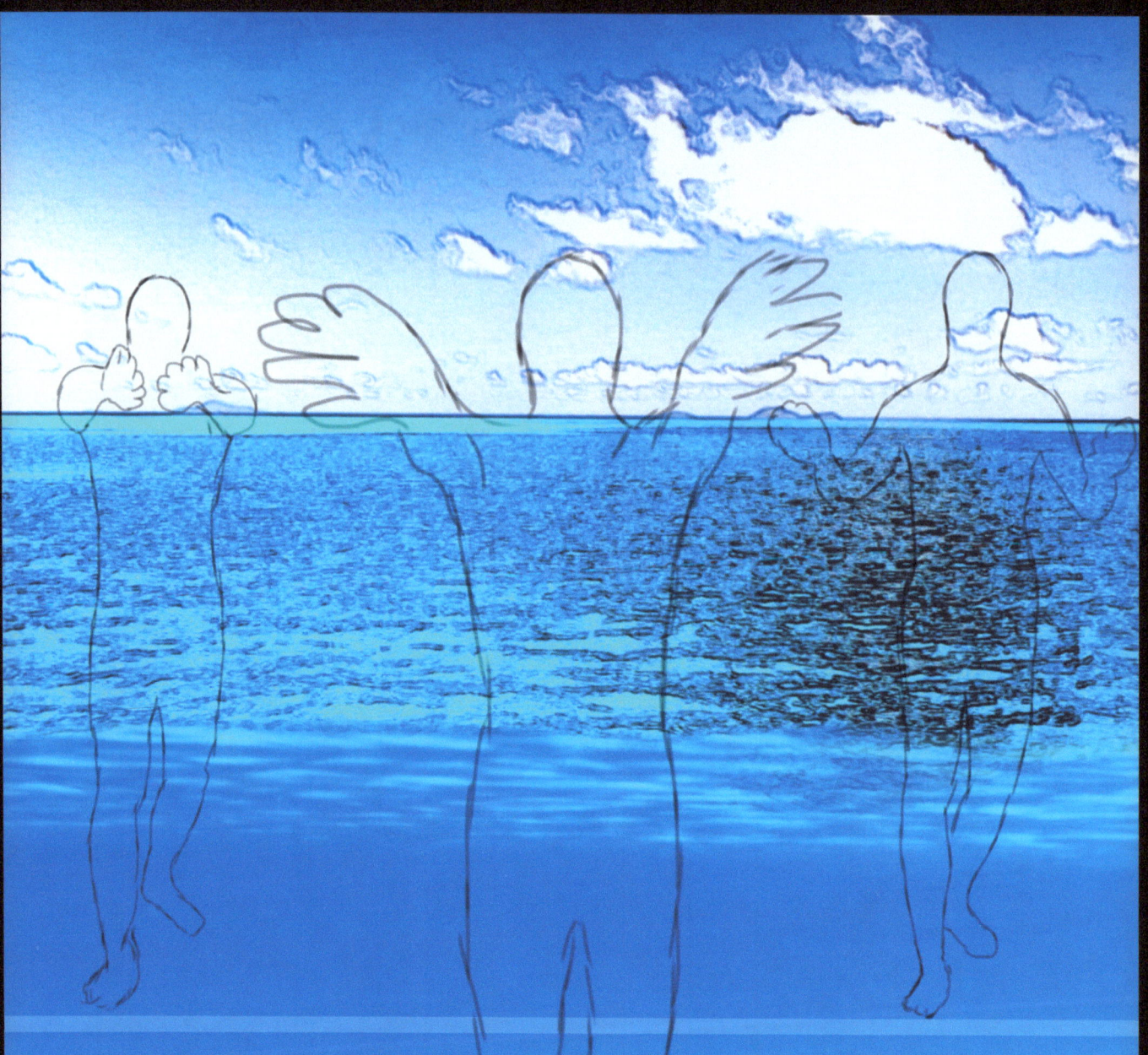

Water at chest level. Arms straight in front, hands facing out, arc your arm to your side. Now arc your arms front with hands facing inward.

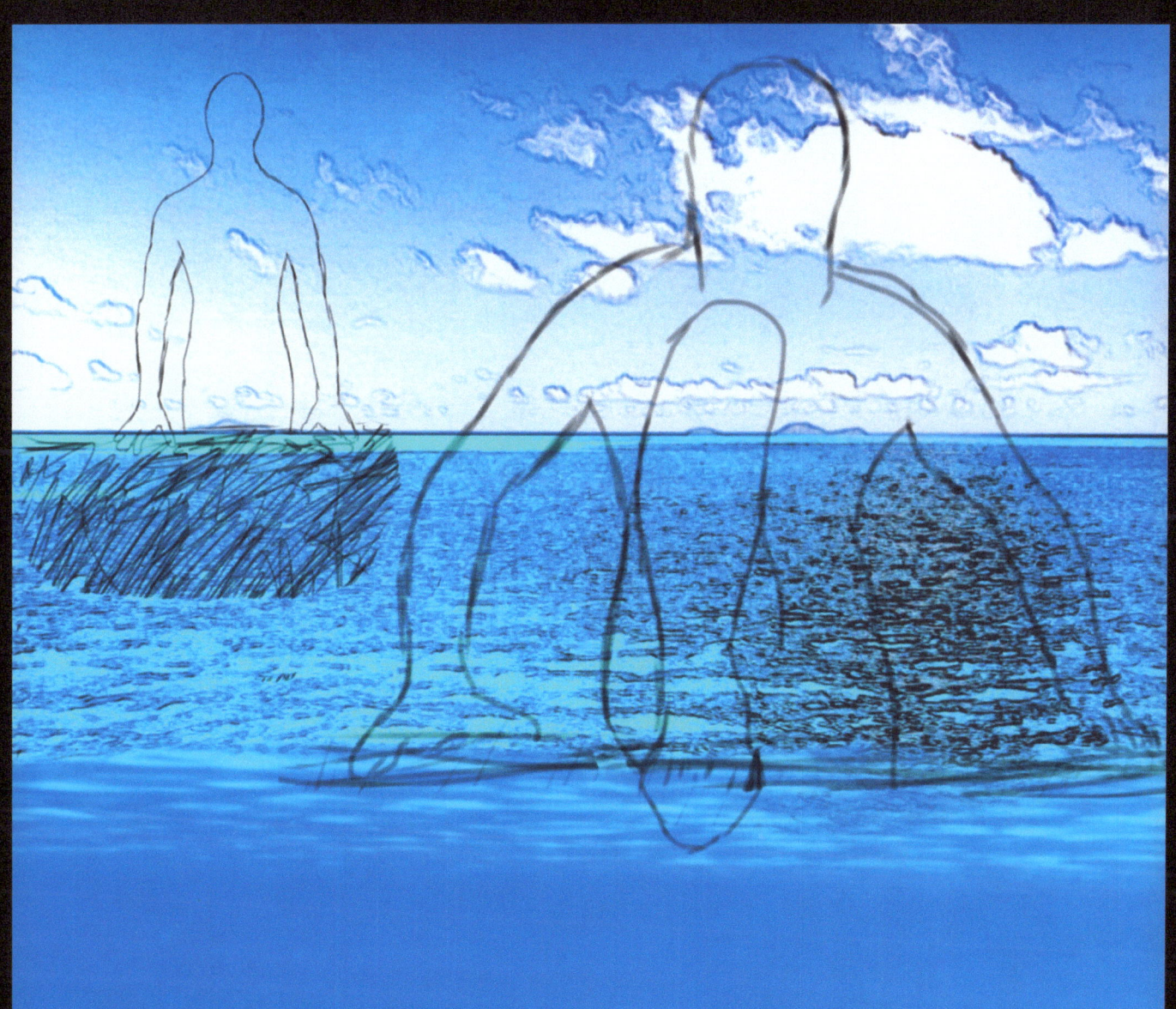

Water at any level. The deeper the water, the harder the move. Hand on the edge of standing pool platform and push yourself up until your arm is straight, then walk up to the platform. Back walk into the pool. Repeat with the other leg.

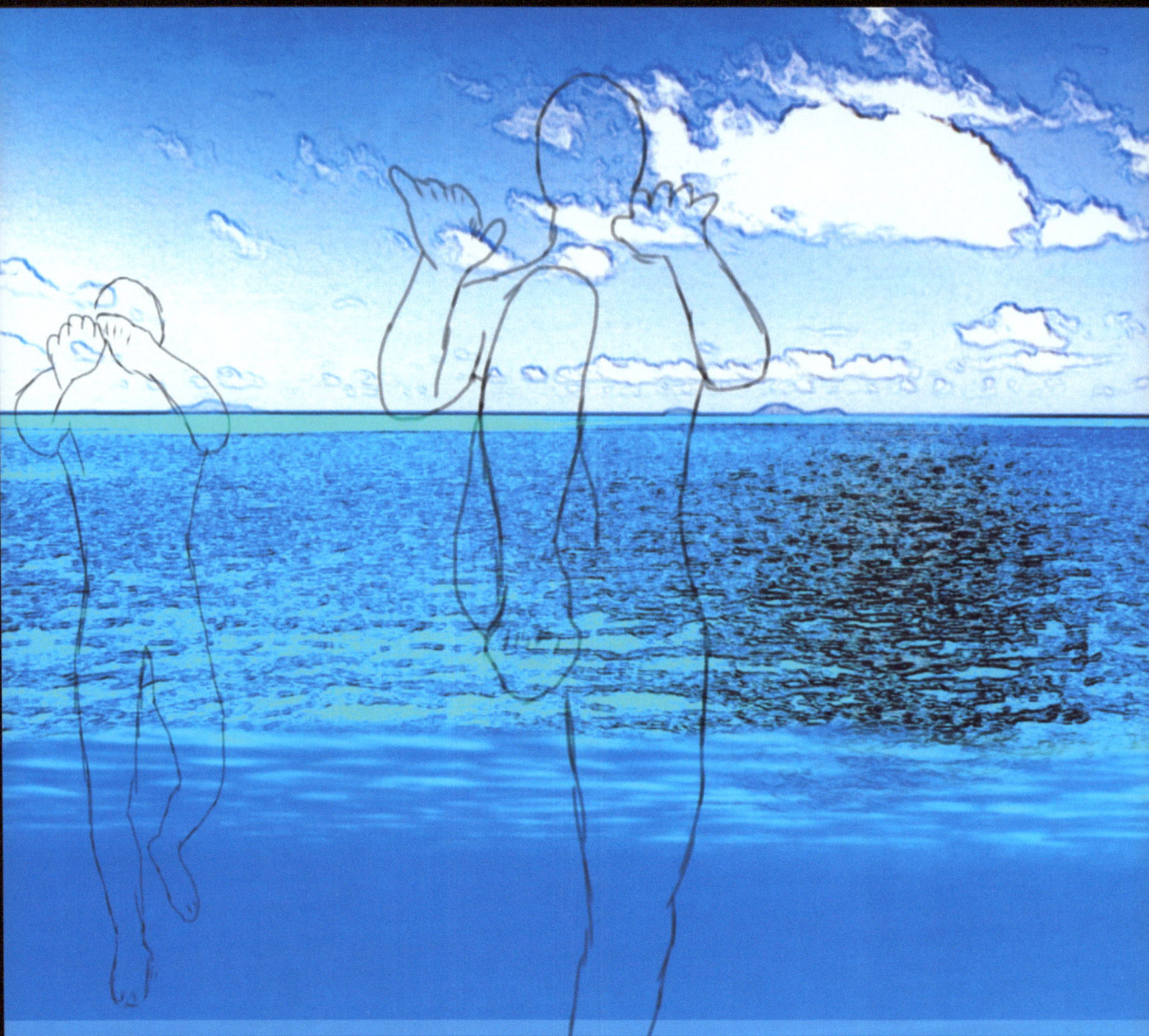

Water at chest level. Holding your hands together straight, arms straight swing to one side. While coming back to center you will come to your chest and then push your hands straight in front of you just below the surface. You will open your hands facing downwards lifting it out of water while doing a Muay Thai Kick.

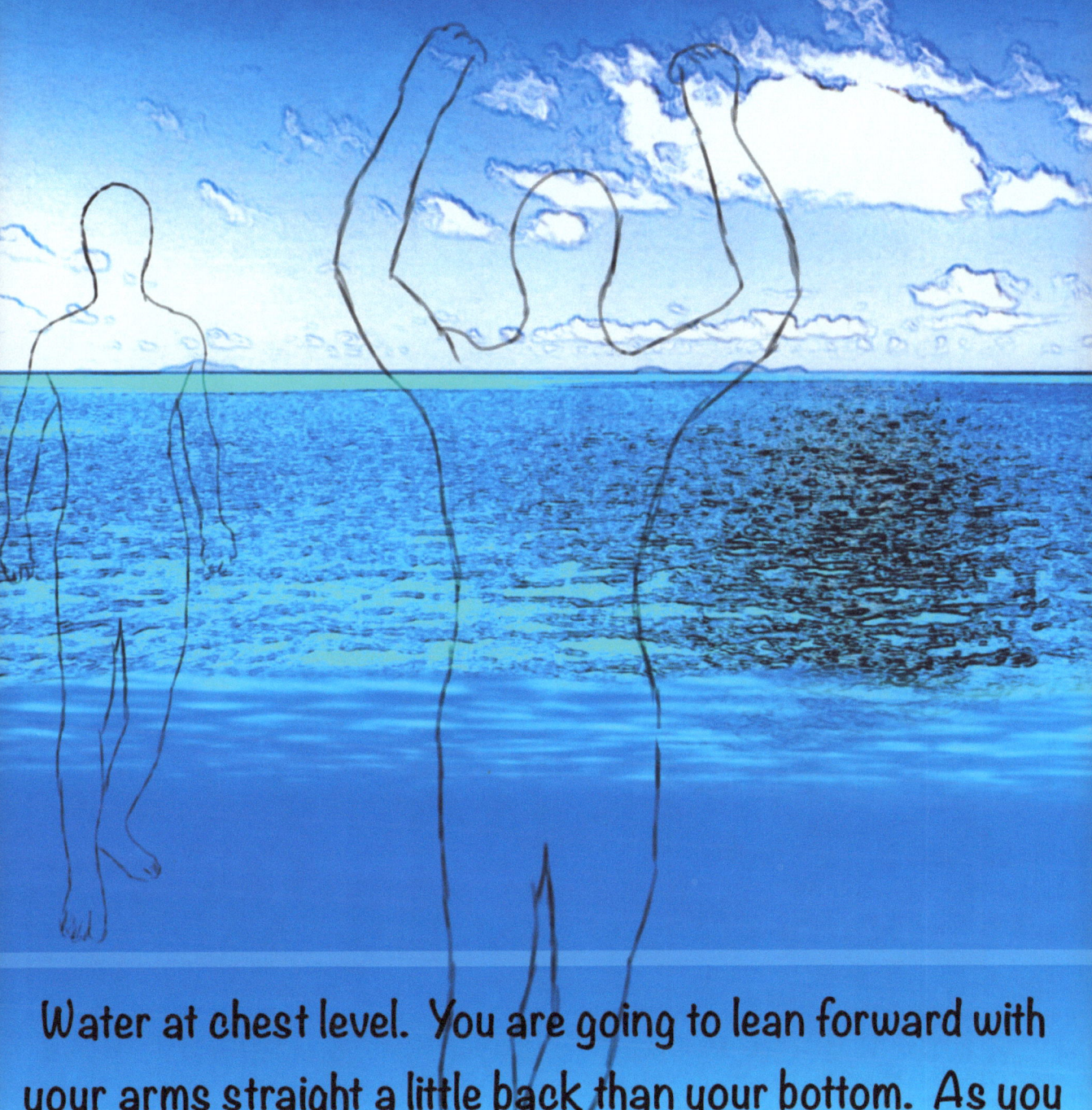

Water at chest level. You are going to lean forward with your arms straight a little back than your bottom. As you walk forward, you will swing your straight arms forward keeping your hands facing forward and up until your hands clears the surface. Now do the opposite motion to propel yourself forward.

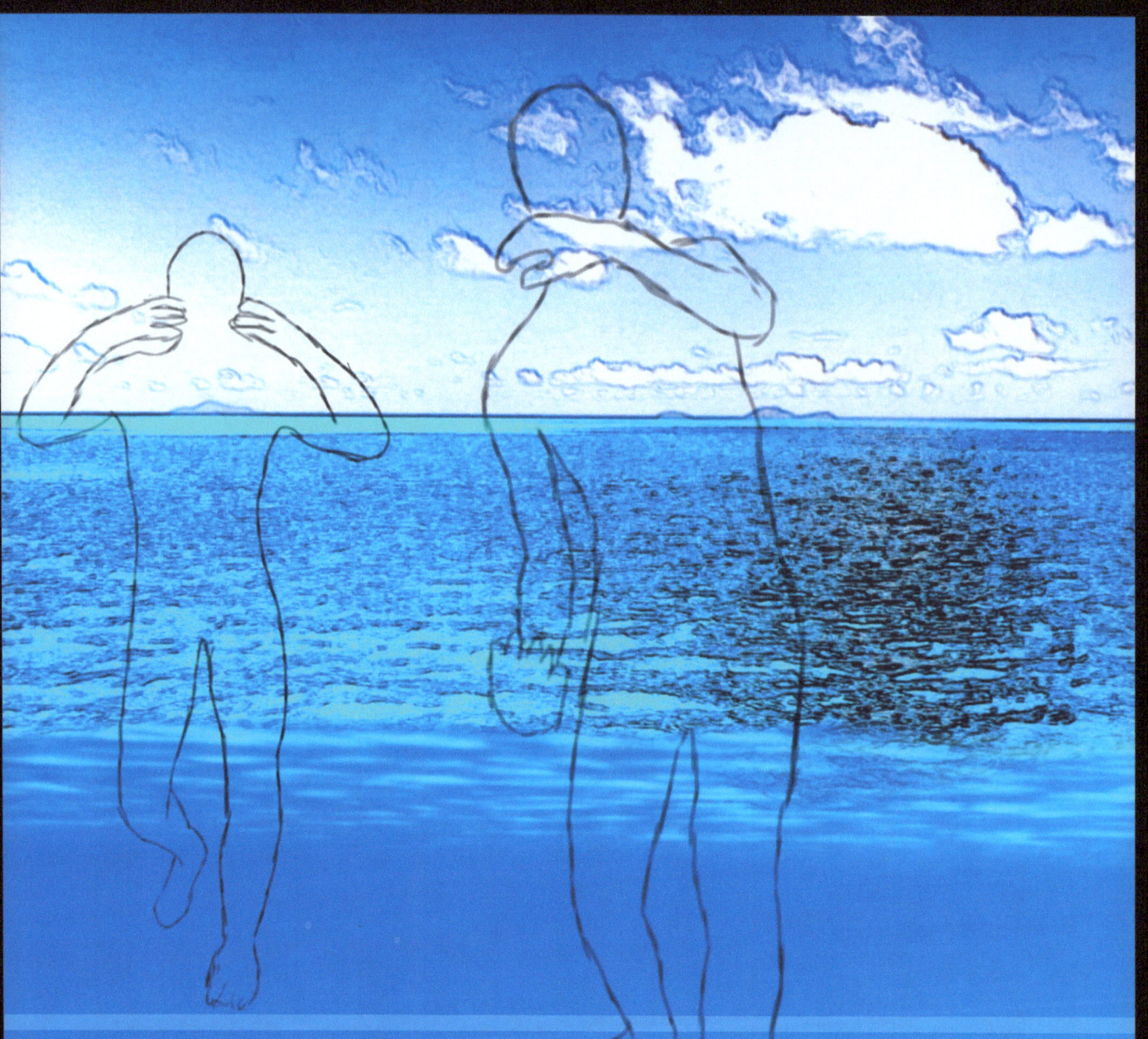

Water at chest level. Do a hug, then do a bowling move with your legs planted untill your hand hit the surface. Switch sides.

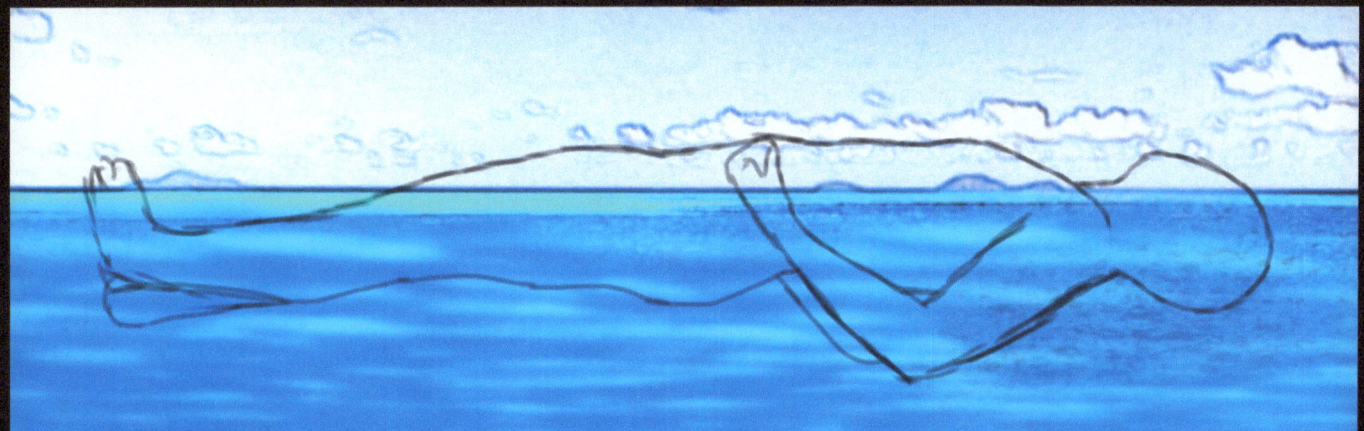

Water at the deepest. This is the most important move of Water Kung Fu. The goal of this move is to reach nirvana. It helps to wear ear putty so you don't get nauseated. This move is to be done at the end of phase 2 or 3 to let you tighten your muscles, strengthen your neck, shoulders and back while doing breathing and meditation exercises. This is also an excellent move for substituting the dragon flag to tone those six packs. This is the only move that doesn't follow the 7 minute workout and 3 minute rest procedure. Instead you will do the Chi Float for 30 minutes. Don't worry if you can't do the float properly for 30 minutes at first. You can use your hands and legs to help keep your self at the float position. The Chi Float position is a straight back float position with your arms on your side with hands closed, hard breath in, head back while you tightening all muscles in your body as long as you can hold your breath while trying to elevate your lower body and legs as much as you can to the water surface. Breath out, repeat. At no time are you allowed your legs or lower body to tilt more than ten degree downwards. After 15 to 20 minutes of this you should able to reach nirvana and you have reached the goal of Water Kung Fu conditioning and for the next 10 to 15 minutes you should be in a meditative mode. During those last 10 to 15 minutes your body will recover to a point that now you can do some extra ordinary stuffs if you want. I end the float with a dead men's float with hands on the side of my head in a fetal position to relax my neck and back. I also do about 10 minutes of water yoga stretches to finish off.

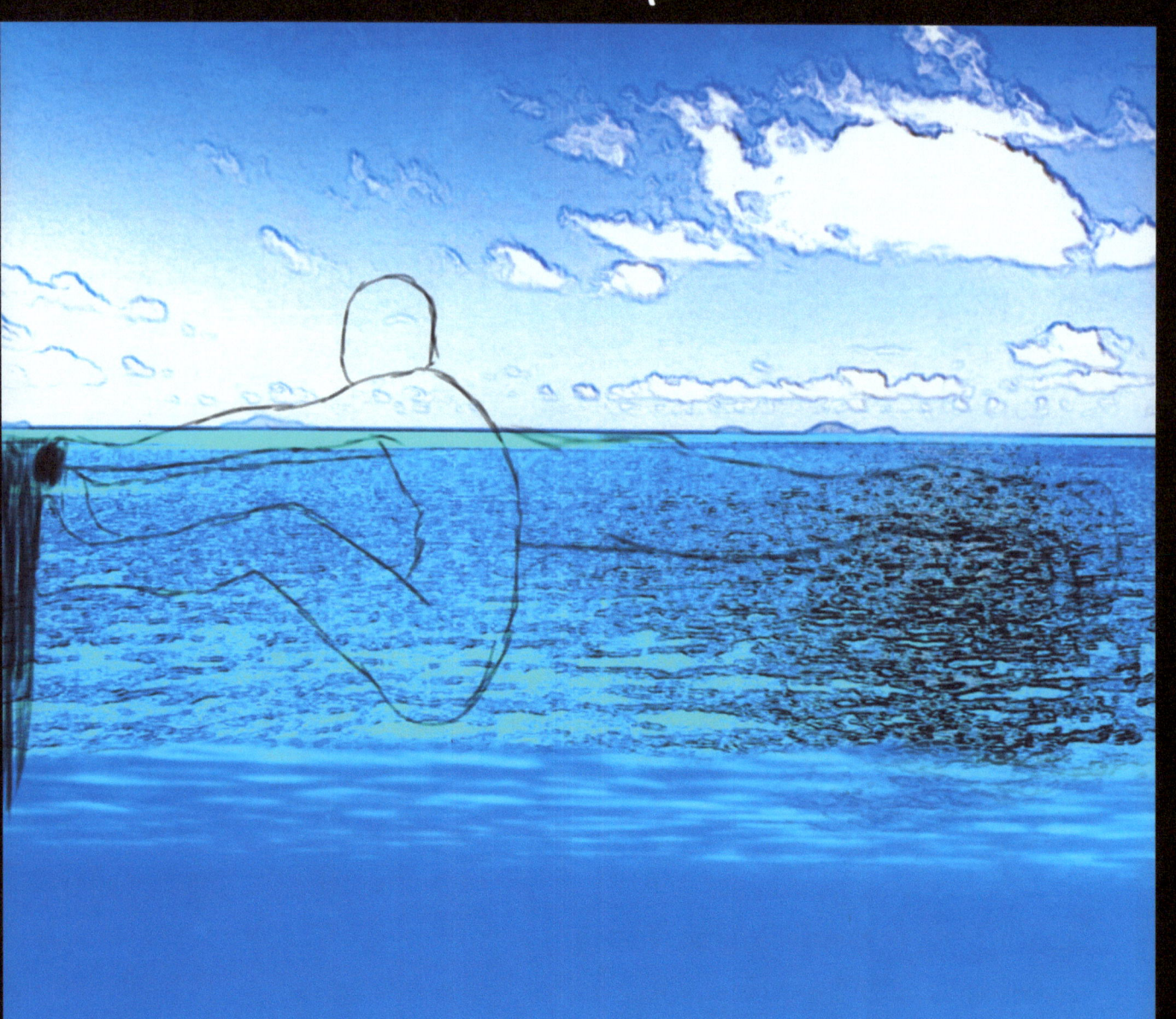

Water at the deepest level. Hold onto the handle bar on the side of the pool. Arms parallel to the water. Feet on pool side while legs are bent. Push with your legs untill your whole body is straight facing down. Now use your arms and body muscles to come back to the initial position as fast as you can.

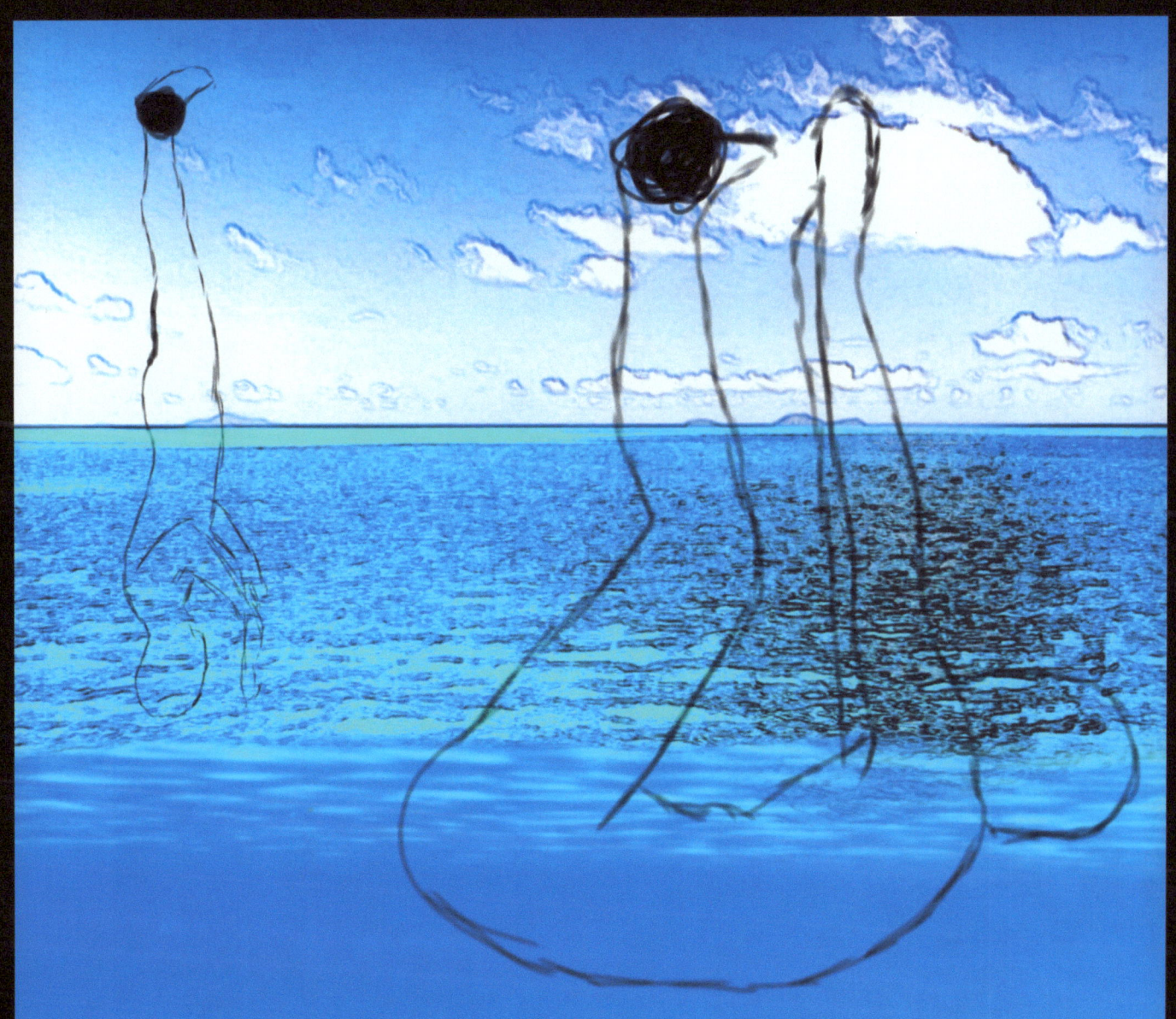

While hanging upside down on the center poll straight making sure your head is above water and your hands submerged in water. Grab water with both of your hands and bring it over the poll. In the right conditions, this will make a rainbow.

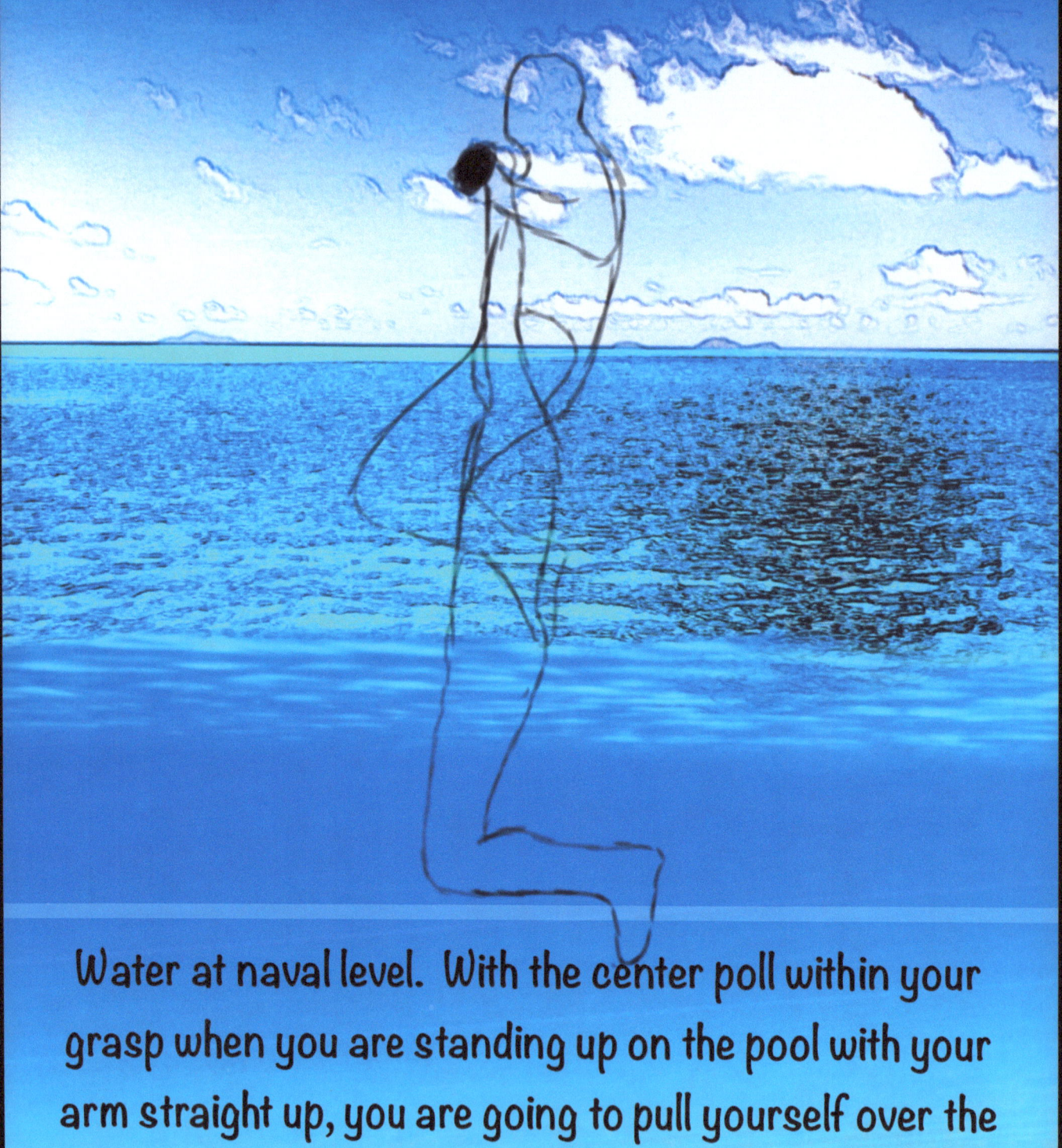

Water at naval level. With the center poll within your grasp when you are standing up on the pool with your arm straight up, you are going to pull yourself over the bar. Ideally you should do this with muscle ups, but anyway you can get over the bar is acceptable even if you have to use your legs.

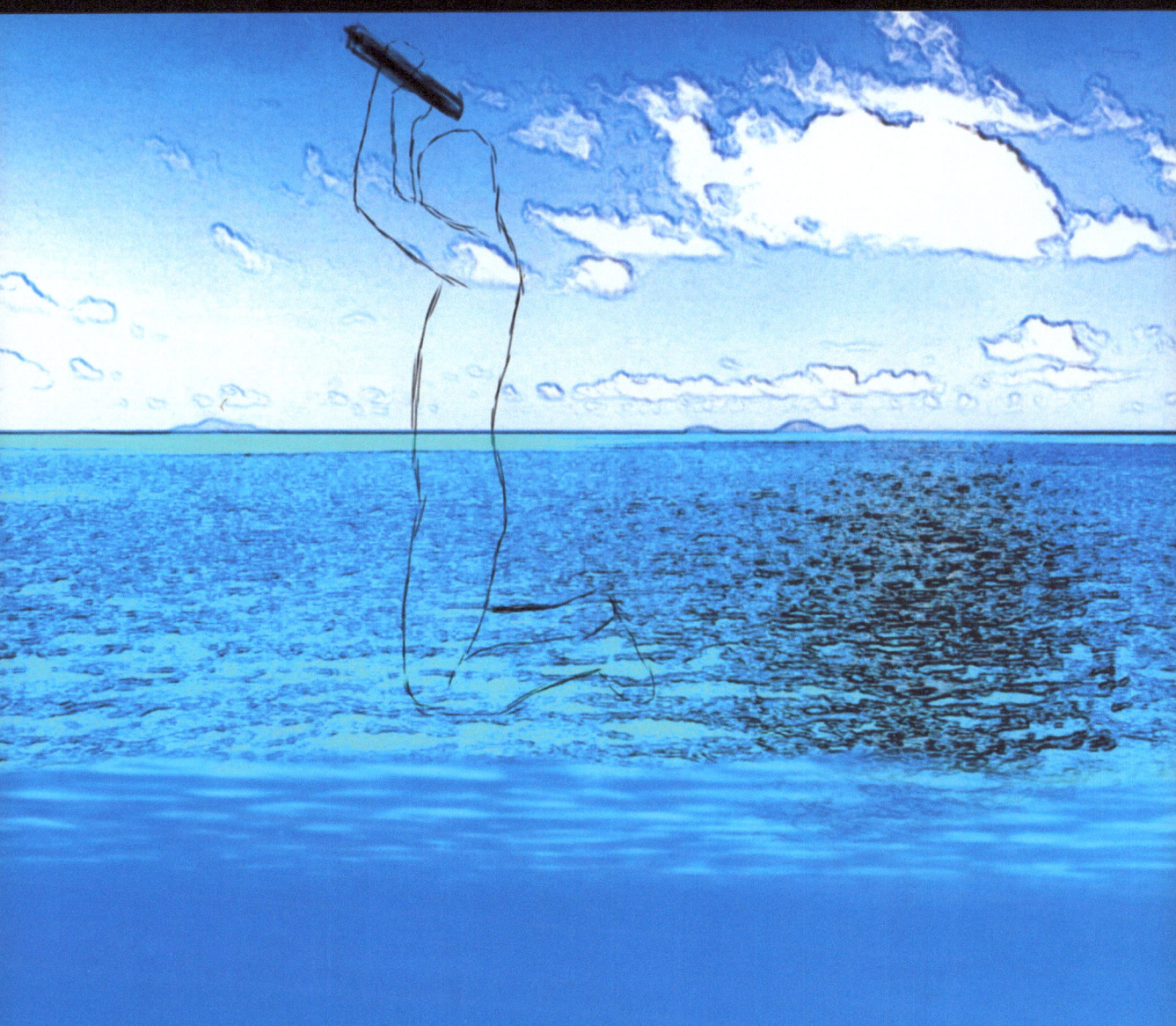

With the center poll at a height when you hang on it arms straight, the water touching your knee, you will not touch the water during the whole move. At no point will your main body or more than two extremities can touch the poll.

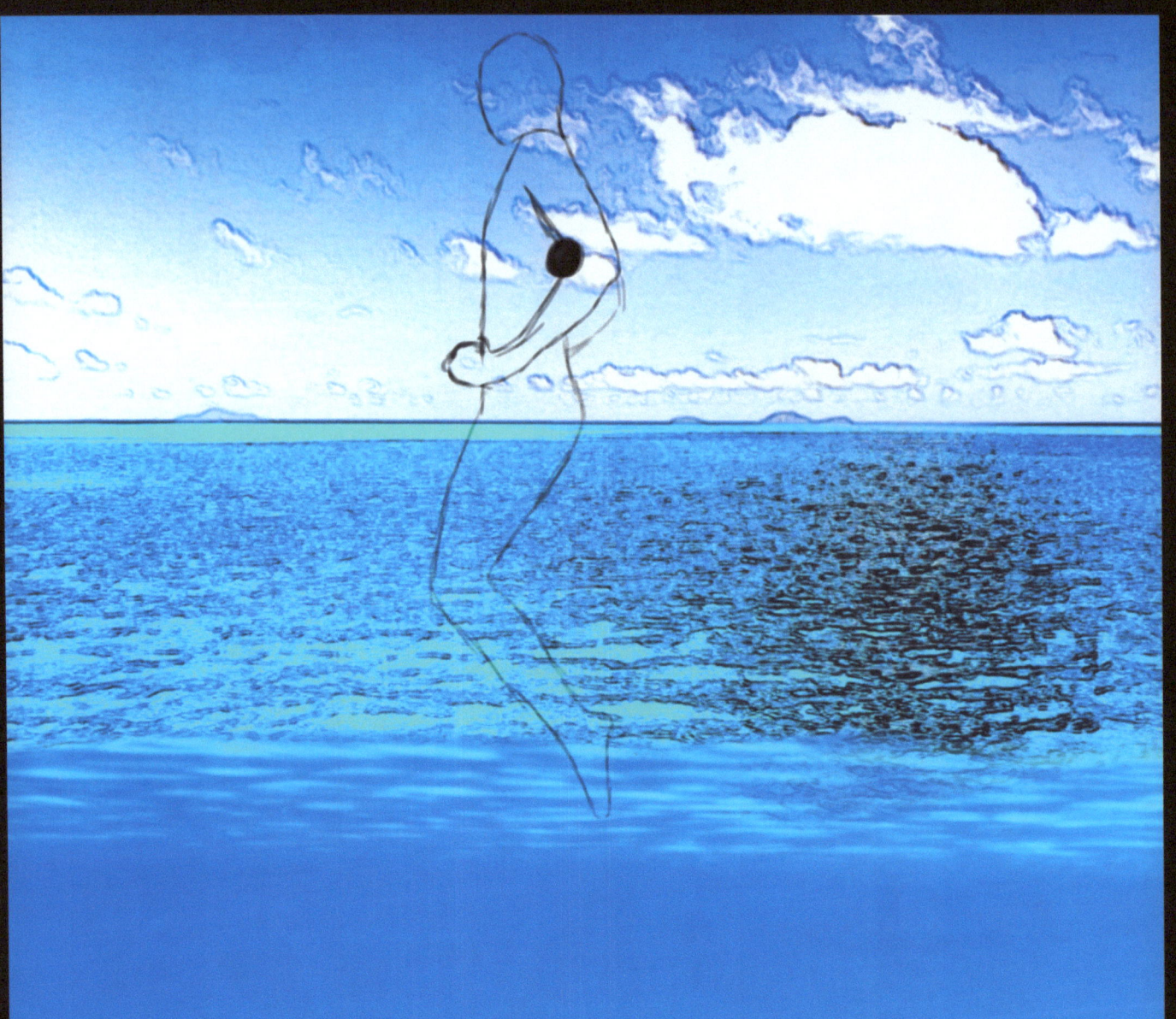

With both crooks of your elbow holding the center poll while your body hanging straight down, the water should be ankle deep. Now using your body and legs as an engine, make yourself spin on the rotating poll.

www.ingramcontent.com/pod-product-compliance
Lightning Source LLC
Chambersburg PA
CBHW041831280526
45792CB00006B/2053